Contents

Introduction

Understanding Diabetes and Weight Loss

Diabetes is a chronic disease that develops when the body struggles to control blood sugar levels. The two main varieties of diabetes are type 1 and type 2.

The immune system of the body targets and kills the cells in the pancreas that make insulin in type 1 diabetes, an autoimmune condition. Insulin is a hormone that helps regulate blood sugar levels by allowing glucose (a type of sugar) to enter cells and be used for energy. Without enough insulin, glucose builds up in the blood, leading to high blood sugar levels (also known as hyperglycemia).

Type 2 diabetes, on the other hand, is a metabolic disorder characterized by the body's inability to properly use insulin. This is known as insulin resistance. In people with type 2 diabetes, the pancreas may not produce enough insulin or the body may not effectively use the insulin it does produce. This can also lead to high blood sugar levels.

Weight loss can be an important part of managing diabetes, especially for people with type 2 diabetes. Losing excess weight can help improve insulin sensitivity and reduce the risk of complications such as heart disease and stroke. However, weight loss can be challenging, especially if you have diabetes.

Several strategies can help people with diabetes lose weight and improve their blood sugar control. These include:

Eating a healthy diet: This means choosing foods that are low in calories, saturated fat, and added sugars, and high in nutrients like fiber, protein, and healthy fats.

Getting regular physical activity: Aim for at least 150 minutes of moderate-intensity exercise or 75 minutes of vigorous-intensity exercise per week.

Monitoring blood sugar levels: Checking blood sugar levels regularly can help you understand how different foods and activities affect your blood sugar and make any necessary adjustments.

Working with a healthcare team: Your healthcare team can provide support and guidance to help you manage your diabetes and reach your weight loss goals.

It's important to note that weight loss is not always easy and may require a combination of lifestyle changes and medication. Working closely with a healthcare team can help you develop a plan that is tailored to your specific needs and goals.

Grace had been living with type 2 diabetes for several years. Despite taking medication and trying to eat a healthy diet, her blood sugar levels remained high and she struggled with excess weight. She was tired of feeling sluggish and worried about the long-term health consequences of her condition.

One day, Grace decided that she had had enough. She was determined to take control of her health and reverse her diabetes. She started by talking to her doctor and nutritionist about her goals. They helped her create a meal plan that focused on whole, unprocessed foods and limited added sugars and unhealthy fats.

Grace also committed to exercising regularly. She started walking every day and gradually increased the intensity and duration of her workouts. As she stuck to her healthy eating and exercise plan, she noticed a dramatic improvement in her energy levels and blood sugar control.

After just a few months, Grace was thrilled to see that her blood sugar levels were within a normal range. She had lost a significant amount of weight and was no longer taking diabetes medication. She felt empowered and grateful for the positive changes she had made in her life.

Grace's story is a testament to the fact that with the right diet and lifestyle changes, it is possible to reverse type 2 diabetes and improve overall health.

The Importance of a Healthy Diet for Diabetes Management

A healthy diet is an essential component of diabetes management. Proper nutrition can help individuals with diabetes better control their blood sugar levels, maintain a healthy weight, and reduce their risk of complications such as heart disease and nerve damage.

Eating a balanced diet that is rich in fruits, vegetables, whole grains, and lean proteins can help individuals with diabetes manage their blood sugar levels and maintain good overall health. It is also important to limit the intake of added sugars, saturated and trans fats, and sodium, as these can contribute to the development of complications.

In addition to following a healthy diet, individuals with diabetes should also pay attention to the portion sizes of the foods they eat, as well as the timing of their meals. Spreading out meals and snacks evenly throughout the day, and consuming them at regular intervals, can help regulate blood sugar levels and prevent large fluctuations.

Working with a registered dietitian or a healthcare provider can help develop a personalized nutrition plan that takes into account an individual's unique needs, preferences, and medical history.

In summary, a healthy diet is a crucial aspect of diabetes management and can help individuals with diabetes better control their blood sugar levels, maintain a healthy weight, and reduce their risk of complications.

Week 1: Getting Started

Day 1: Meal Planning and Grocery Shopping

On day 1 of your meal planning and grocery shopping, there are a few steps you can follow to help make the process as efficient and successful as possible:

1. Make a list: Start by making a list of all the meals and snacks you will need for the week. Consider the number of people you are feeding, your schedule, and any dietary restrictions or preferences. You can use this list to help you plan out your meals and create a grocery list.

2. Check your pantry and fridge: Before you head to the store, take a look at what you already have on hand. This can help you avoid buying duplicates or items that you don't need.

3. Make a plan: Once you have your list and know what you already have, it's time to plan out your meals for the week. Consider the number of meals you will need to prepare each day, and try to balance your meals with a variety of protein sources, fruits, vegetables, and whole grains.

4. Shop smart: When you go to the store, try to stick to your list as much as possible. Avoid impulse

purchases and look for sales or discounts on items you regularly use. You can also consider buying in bulk or shopping at stores that offer lower prices on healthy options.

5. Organize your groceries: When you get home, take the time to properly store your groceries. This can help them stay fresh and prevent waste.

By following these steps, you can make the process of meal planning and grocery shopping more efficient and effective, which can help you stay on track with your healthy eating goals.

Day 2: Breakfast Ideas

On day 2, here are some healthy breakfast ideas to help you start your day off right:

1. Overnight oats: Combine rolled oats, Greek yogurt, milk, and your favorite fruit in a jar or container. Let it sit in the fridge overnight, and in the morning, you'll have a quick and easy breakfast that is high in protein and fiber.

Avocado toast: Toast a slice of whole grain bread, and then mash half an avocado on top. Add a sprinkle of salt and pepper, and top with a fried egg or sliced tomato for added flavor and nutrition.

2. Smoothie bowl: Blend your favorite fruits, a handful of greens, and some protein-rich Greek yogurt or milk for a nourishing breakfast bowl. Top with your choice of nuts, seeds, and fruit for added crunch and flavor.

3. Breakfast burrito: Fill a whole grain tortilla with scrambled eggs, black beans, diced tomato, and avocado. Top with a sprinkle of cheese and a dollop of salsa for added flavor.

4. Egg muffins: Preheat your oven to 350 degrees. Place an egg in each of the muffin cups after greasing the pan. Add your favorite toppings such as diced vegetables, cheese, or cooked sausage. Until the eggs are set, bake for 15 to 20 minutes.

These are just a few ideas to get you started, but the possibilities for a healthy breakfast are endless. Experiment with different ingredients and see what works best for you.

Day 3: Lunch Ideas

Here are some lunch ideas for day 3

Grilled chicken salad: Grill some chicken breasts and slice them into thin strips. Toss with mixed greens, cherry tomatoes, cucumber, red onion, and your choice of dressing.

Quinoa and black bean burrito bowls: Cook quinoa and mix with black beans, corn, diced tomatoes, and diced bell peppers. Serve over a bed of lettuce and top with avocado, cheese, and salsa.

Tuna salad sandwich: Mix canned tuna with mayonnaise, diced celery, and diced onions. Spread the mixture onto slices of bread and top with lettuce and tomato.

Turkey and avocado wrap: Spread mashed avocado onto a tortilla, and top with sliced turkey, lettuce, tomato, and a drizzle of ranch dressing. Roll up the tortilla and slice it in half to serve.

Greek yogurt and fruit parfait: Layer Greek yogurt, sliced strawberries, and granola in a jar or bowl. Repeat the layers until the jar is full and top with a sprinkle of honey.

Veggie and hummus wrap: Spread hummus onto a tortilla and top with sliced cucumbers, bell peppers, and carrots. Roll up the tortilla and slice it in half to serve.

Peanut butter and jelly sandwich: Spread peanut butter and jelly onto slices of bread and serve with a side of carrot sticks and cherry tomatoes.

Grilled cheese and tomato soup: Make a classic grilled cheese sandwich using your favorite bread and cheese. Serve with a cup of tomato soup on the side.

Day 4: Dinner Ideas

Here are some dinner ideas for Day 4

1. Grilled chicken with a salad: Grilled chicken is a healthy and flavorful option for dinner. Serve it with a salad of mixed greens, cherry tomatoes, and your favorite dressing.

2. Spaghetti with meatballs: A classic dinner option, spaghetti with meatballs is sure to be a hit with the whole family. You can make your meatballs or use store-bought ones to save time.

3. Quiche with a side of roasted vegetables: Quiche is a versatile dish that can be filled with all sorts of ingredients, such as cheese, vegetables, and meat. For

a complete supper, serve it with a side of roasted veggies.

4. Black bean burritos: These burritos are easy to make and filled with protein-rich black beans, cheese, and your choice of vegetables. Serve with a side of guacamole and sour cream for dipping.

5. Salmon with roasted potatoes and asparagus: This dinner is a little more upscale, but it's still easy to make. Grill or bake the salmon, and roast some potatoes and asparagus in the oven. Top it off with a squeeze of lemon juice and a sprinkle of herbs.

Day 5: Snack Ideas

Here are some snack ideas for Day 5

1. Apple slices with peanut butter: This simple snack is a great combination of sweet and savory. Slice up an apple and dip the pieces into a spoonful of peanut butter for a satisfying snack.

2. Hummus with veggies: Hummus is a healthy and tasty dip that goes well with a variety of vegetables. Cut up some carrots, bell peppers, and celery and serve them with a bowl of hummus for dipping.

3. Hard-boiled eggs: Hard-boiled eggs are a convenient and protein-rich snack that can be easily prepared in advance. Sprinkle them with a little bit of salt and pepper for added flavor.

4. Greek yogurt with berries: Greek yogurt is a high-protein snack that's also good for your gut. Top it with a handful of fresh berries for a burst of flavor.

5. Cheese and crackers: This classic snack combination is always a hit. Choose a variety of cheeses and crackers to mix and match flavors.

Remember to choose snacks that are balanced and provide nutrients to keep you satisfied between meals.

Day 6: Exercise and Physical Activity

Here are some ideas for exercise and physical activity on Day 6

1. Go for a walk or jog: Taking a walk or going for a jog is a simple and enjoyable way to get some physical activity. Head to a local park or trail for a change of scenery.

2. Join a group fitness class: Many gyms and community centers offer group fitness classes, such

as yoga, Pilates, and Zumba. These classes can be a fun way to get in a workout while also being social.

3. Do a home workout: There are plenty of workout routines that can be done at home with minimal equipment. Look online for videos or tutorials that suit your fitness level and goals.
4. Go cycling: If you have a bike, consider going for a ride through your neighborhood or a nearby park. This is a great way to get in some cardio while also enjoying the outdoors.
5. Play a sport: Engage in a sport you enjoy, such as basketball, tennis, or soccer. This can be a fun and competitive way to get in some physical activity.

Remember to choose an activity that you enjoy and that fits into your schedule. It's crucial to pay attention to your body's signals and take breaks when necessary.

Day 7: Tracking Progress and Staying Motivated

Welcome to Day 7 of your journey! By now, you've probably been working on your goals for a week and you may be starting to feel the weight of the task at hand. It's important to keep track of your progress and stay motivated to stay on track. Here are some tips for tracking progress and staying motivated:

1. Set small, achievable goals: It's important to set realistic goals that you can accomplish in a short amount of time. Your motivation will remain high as a result of this and you'll feel more accomplished.

2. Keep a record of your progress: Whether you use a planner, a spreadsheet, or a simple notebook, it's important to keep track of what you've accomplished. Seeing your progress will help you stay motivated and give you a sense of accomplishment.

3. Celebrate your victories: No matter how small, it's important to take a moment to celebrate your victories. This could be as simple as acknowledging your progress or treating yourself to something special.

4. Find a support system: Surround yourself with people who will support you and encourage you to stay on track. This could be friends, family, or a coach or mentor.

5. Stay positive: It's important to stay positive, even when things aren't going as planned. Remind yourself of your long-term goals and the progress you've made so far.

Remember, progress takes time and it's normal to encounter setbacks along the way. The important thing is to keep moving forward and stay motivated to achieve your goals.

Week 2: Incorporating More Plant-Based Foods

Welcome to Week 2 of incorporating more plant-based foods into your diet! By now, you should have a good understanding of the benefits of plant-based eating and have started experimenting with some new recipes and ingredients. This week, we'll focus on expanding your plant-based repertoire and finding ways to incorporate more plant-based foods into your meals and snacks.

Here are some ideas for getting started:
Experiment with different types of plant-based protein

1. sources: There are so many options beyond just beans and tofu. Try incorporating lentils, chickpeas, nuts, and seeds into your meals. You can also try using plant-based protein powders in smoothies or as a base for homemade energy bars.

2. Go meatless one day a week: Choose a day of the week to go entirely meatless. This can be a great way to try out new plant-based recipes and get creative with your meals.

3. Add more vegetables to your meals: Vegetables are an important part of a plant-based diet and can be incorporated into just about any meal. Try adding roasted vegetables to pasta dishes, using zucchini

noodles in place of regular noodles, or packing a salad full of different types of greens.

4. Try plant-based dairy alternatives: If you're trying to reduce your intake of animal products, plant-based dairy alternatives can be a great option. There are many types of plant-based kinds of milk available, including almond, soy, and oat milk. You can also try using plant-based versions of cheese and yogurt.

5. Make a meal plan: Planning out your meals for the week can help you stay on track with your plant-based goals. Make a list of the plant-based meals and snacks you want to eat and shop for the ingredients in advance. This will make it easier to stick to your plan and make healthier choices.

Remember to be patient and give yourself time to adjust to this new way of eating. It can take some time to get used to new flavors and textures, but the more you practice, the easier it will become. Keep trying new recipes and have fun experimenting with plant-based foods.

Day 8: Plant-Based Protein Sources

Welcome to Day 8 of incorporating more plant-based foods into your diet! Today, we'll be focusing on plant-based protein sources. It's important to include protein in your diet as it helps to build and repair tissues, produce enzymes and hormones, and support a healthy immune system.

Here are some great plant-based protein sources to add to your meals and snacks:

1. Beans and legumes: These include lentils, chickpeas, kidney beans, black beans, and more. They are a great source of protein and fiber and can be easily added to soups, salads, and pasta dishes.

2. Tofu: Made from soybeans, tofu is a fantastic source of protein. It is very versatile and can be used in a variety of dishes, including stir-fries, soups, and curries.

3. Nuts and seeds are a fantastic source of protein and good fats.. Some options include almonds, cashews, peanuts, sunflower seeds, and pumpkin seeds. They can be eaten on their own as a snack or added to salads, oatmeal, and baked goods.

4. Plant-based protein powders: These can be a convenient way to add protein to smoothies or

homemade energy bars. Some options include pea protein, hemp protein, and soy protein.

5. Grains: Whole grains like quinoa, bulgur, and farro are also a good source of protein. They can be used as a base for salads or added to soups and stews.

Remember to include a variety of protein sources in your diet to ensure you are getting all the essential amino acids. Have fun experimenting with these plant-based protein sources and incorporating them into your meals.

Day 9: Incorporating More Fruits and Vegetables

Welcome to Day 9 of incorporating more plant-based foods into your diet! Today, we'll be focusing on ways to add more fruits and vegetables to your meals and snacks. Fruits and vegetables are an important part of a healthy, plant-based diet as they provide essential nutrients, fiber, and antioxidants.

Here are some ideas for incorporating more fruits and vegetables into your diet:

1. Make a smoothie: Smoothies are a great way to pack in a lot of fruits and vegetables in one sitting. Try

using a base of leafy greens like spinach or kale and adding in a variety of fruits like berries, bananas, and mango. You can also add in some protein powder or nut butter for added staying power.

2. Add vegetables to your meals: Try adding roasted or sautéed vegetables to your pasta dishes, grain bowls, and soups. You can also use vegetables like zucchini and eggplant as a pasta substitute or try making a stir-fry with a variety of vegetables.

3. Snack on fruits and vegetables: Keep a variety of cut-up fruits and vegetables on hand for quick and easy snacking. Some options include carrot sticks, cherry tomatoes, grapes, and sliced apples.

4. Make a salad: Salads are a great way to get a lot of vegetables in one meal. Try using a variety of greens like kale, spinach, and arugula and adding in a variety of colorful vegetables like bell peppers, cherry tomatoes, and beets. You can also add in some protein like tofu or chickpeas to make it a more substantial meal.

5. Try new fruits and vegetables: Don't be afraid to try new fruits and vegetables. There are so many different types available, and trying new things can be a fun and exciting way to mix up your meals.

Remember to aim for at least 5 servings of fruits and vegetables per day. They can be eaten raw, cooked, or frozen, so there are many options for incorporating them into your diet. Have fun experimenting with different ways to add more fruits and vegetables to your meals.

Day 10: Plant-Based Meal Ideas

Welcome to Day 10 of incorporating more plant-based foods into your diet! By now, you should have a good understanding of the benefits of plant-based eating and have started experimenting with some new recipes and ingredients. Today, we'll be focusing on some delicious plant-based meal ideas to try out.

Here are some ideas to get you started:

1. Vegan stir-fry: Stir-fries are a quick and easy way to get a lot of vegetables into your diet. Try using a base of brown rice or quinoa and adding in a variety of vegetables like bell peppers, broccoli, and carrots. You can also add in some tofu or tempeh for protein.
2. Veggie burger: There are many different types of veggie burgers available at most grocery stores or

you can make your own using beans, lentils, or grains as a base. Serve the burger on a whole grain bun with your favorite toppings like avocado, tomato, and lettuce.

3. Vegan pasta dish: Pasta is a great base for a plant-based meal. Try using a tomato-based sauce and adding in a variety of vegetables like bell peppers, zucchini, and eggplant. You can also add in some protein like tofu or tempeh.

4. Vegetable quesadilla: Quesadillas are a quick and easy meal that can be made plant-based by using a tortilla and filling it with a variety of vegetables like bell peppers, onions, and mushrooms. You can also add in some plant-based cheese or avocado for added flavor.

5. Vegan grain bowl: Grain bowls are a great way to get a lot of nutrients in one meal. Try using a base of quinoa or brown rice and adding in a variety of vegetables like roasted sweet potatoes, steamed broccoli, and sautéed mushrooms. You can also add in some protein like tofu or tempeh.

Remember to be creative and have fun experimenting with different plant-based ingredients and recipes. There are so many delicious plant-based meals to try, so get creative and enjoy.

Day 11: Substituting Whole Grains for Refined Grains

Welcome to Day 11 of incorporating more plant-based foods into your diet! Today, we'll be focusing on substituting whole grains for refined grains. Whole grains are a great source of nutrients, including fiber, protein, and essential vitamins and minerals. They can also help to lower the risk of heart disease, diabetes, and other chronic diseases.

Here are some tips for incorporating more whole grains into your diet:

1. Choose whole grain bread: Instead of white bread, try using whole grain bread for sandwiches and toast. A whole grain should be the first ingredient on any bread you buy.
2. Use whole grains as a base for salads and grain bowls: Instead of using white rice, try using whole grains like quinoa, farro, or brown rice as a base for

salads and grain bowls. These grains are a great source of protein and can add some variety to your meals.

3. Choose whole grain pasta: Instead of using white pasta, try using whole grain pasta. It is often made from wheat, but can also be made from other grains like quinoa or brown rice.

4. Experiment with different types of whole grains: There are many different types of whole grains to try, including oats, barley, bulgur, and farro. These grains can be used in a variety of dishes, including soups, stews, and salads.

5. Look for whole grain options in packaged foods: When shopping for packaged foods, look for options that are made with whole grains. This includes items like whole grain crackers, cereals, and granola bars.

Remember, it's important to include a variety of whole grains in your diet for optimal health. Try incorporating a few whole grain options into your meals and snacks each day to get the benefits of these nutritious foods.

Remember, it's important to include a variety of whole grains in your diet for optimal health. Try incorporating a few whole grain options into your meals and snacks each day to get the benefits of these nutritious foods.

Day 12: Using Healthy Fats in Cooking and Baking

Welcome to Day 12 of our series on healthy eating! Today, we'll be discussing the importance of using healthy fats in cooking and baking.

It's important to include fats in our diet as they provide a source of energy, help with the absorption of certain vitamins and minerals, and support brain health. However, not all fats are created equal. It's important to choose healthy fats, such as monounsaturated and polyunsaturated fats, over unhealthy ones like trans fats and saturated fats.

Here are some ways to incorporate healthy fats into your cooking and baking:

1. Use olive oil or avocado oil when sautéing or roasting vegetables. These oils are high in monounsaturated fats and have a relatively low smoke point, making them suitable for medium-heat cooking.
2. Swap out butter for coconut oil in baking recipes. Coconut oil is high in saturated fats, but these are the

3. healthy kind that can actually help to raise good cholesterol levels.

4. Add nuts and seeds to your dishes. These are high in polyunsaturated fats and can add flavor and texture to salads, smoothies, and baked goods.

Include fatty fish in your meals. Salmon, tuna, and sardines are all high in omega-3 fatty acids, which have numerous health benefits.

Remember to still consume fats in moderation as they are high in calories. But by including healthy fats in your diet, you can help to support overall health and wellness.

Day 13: Finding Plant-Based Alternatives to Animal Products

Welcome to Day 13 of our series on healthy eating! Today, we'll be discussing plant-based alternatives to animal products.

For those looking to reduce their consumption of animal products or follow a vegetarian or vegan diet, there are many delicious and nutritious plant-based alternatives available. These alternatives can help to provide important nutrients and can be a great way to add variety to your meals.

Here are some plant-based alternatives to common animal products:

1. Tofu and tempeh can be used as a protein source in place of meat. Both are made from soybeans and are high in protein and iron.
2. Legumes, such as lentils, beans, and chickpeas, are also a good source of protein and can be used in place of meat in dishes like soups, stews, and salads.
3. Nutritional yeast is a great plant-based alternative to cheese. It has a cheesy flavor and is high in B-vitamins.
4. Plant-based milks, such as almond milk, soy milk, and oat milk, can be used as a dairy-free alternative to cow's milk.

For a plant-based alternative to eggs, try using a "flax egg" in baking. To make a flax egg, mix together 1 tablespoon of ground flaxseed with 3 tablespoons of water and let it sit for a few minutes to thicken.

By incorporating these plant-based alternatives into your diet, you can still enjoy delicious and satisfying meals while reducing your intake of animal products.

Day 14: Plant-Based Recipe Ideas

Welcome to Day 14 of our series on healthy eating! Today, we'll be sharing some delicious plant-based recipe ideas to help you incorporate more plant-based foods into your diet.

1. Grilled Portobello Mushroom Burgers: Grill portobello mushrooms and serve them on a bun with your choice of toppings, such as avocado, lettuce, tomato, and onion.
2. Spaghetti Squash with Roasted Tomatoes and Garlic: Roast spaghetti squash and top with a sauce made from roasted cherry tomatoes and garlic.
3. Vegetable Stir-Fry: Sauté a variety of vegetables, such as bell peppers, onions, and broccoli, in a wok or large pan. Serve over brown rice or quinoa.
4. Black Bean and Sweet Potato Tacos: Mash black beans and sweet potatoes together and stuff them into

taco shells. Top with shredded lettuce, diced tomatoes, and a drizzle of avocado or cashew cream.

Quinoa and Roasted Vegetable Salad: Roast a variety of vegetables, such as bell peppers, zucchini, and cherry tomatoes, and mix them with cooked quinoa and a vinaigrette dressing.

By incorporating more plant-based foods into your diet, you can enjoy a wide variety of delicious and nutritious meals.

Week 3: Making Healthy Choices When Eating Out

Welcome to Week 3 of our series on healthy eating! Today, we'll be discussing how to make healthy choices when eating out.

Eating out can sometimes be challenging when it comes to maintaining a healthy diet, but it is possible to make healthy choices when dining at restaurants or fast food establishments. Here are some tips to help you make healthier choices when eating out:

Look for restaurants that offer a variety of healthy options, such as salads, grilled chicken or fish, and steamed or roasted vegetables.
Choose grilled, baked, or steamed options over fried items.

Instead of drinking sugary beverages, choose water or unsweetened tea.

Share a meal with a friend or family member or take home leftovers to have for another meal.

Ask for dressing or sauces on the side so that you can control how much you use.

Consider ordering an appetizer as your main meal.

By following these tips, you can still enjoy eating out while making healthier choices. Remember to also be mindful of portion sizes and avoid overeating.

Day 15: Choosing the Right Restaurant

Welcome to Day 15 of our series on healthy eating! Today, we'll be discussing how to choose the right restaurant when eating out.

Eating out can be a convenient and enjoyable experience, but it's important to choose a restaurant that offers healthy options. Here are some tips to help you choose the right restaurant:

Look for restaurants that offer a variety of healthy options, such as salads, grilled chicken or fish, and steamed or roasted vegetables.

Check the menu online before you go to the restaurant. Many restaurants have their menus available online, which can help you to make healthier choices before you even arrive.

Choose a restaurant that uses fresh ingredients and prepares dishes in a healthy way, such as grilling or baking instead of frying.

Consider the atmosphere and ambiance of the restaurant. A more upscale or fine dining establishment may be more likely to offer healthier options than a fast food chain.

Look for restaurants that offer options for dietary restrictions, such as vegetarian, vegan, or gluten-free options.

By following these tips, you can choose a restaurant that offers healthy options and helps you to maintain a healthy diet while eating out

Day 16: Selecting Healthy Options on the Menu

Welcome to Day 16 of our healthy living journey! Today, we will be focusing on selecting healthy options when dining out or ordering from a menu.

Eating out can be a fun and enjoyable experience, but it can also be a challenge if you are trying to maintain a healthy diet. With so many tempting options available, it can be easy to fall into the trap of choosing unhealthy meals. However, with a little planning and some mindful decision making, it is possible to enjoy dining out while still making healthy choices.

Here are some tips to help you select healthy options when dining out:

Look for options that are high in protein and fiber: These nutrients help keep you feeling full and satisfied. Choose dishes that include vegetables, beans, legumes, and lean protein sources such as grilled chicken or fish.

Choose dishes that are grilled, baked, or steamed: These cooking methods tend to be healthier than fried options.

Avoid dishes that are heavy on the sauce: Sauces, dressings, and gravies can add a lot of extra calories and fat to your meal. Opt for dishes that are served with minimal sauce or ask for sauces on the side so you can control how much you use.

Don't be afraid to make substitutions: Many restaurants are willing to accommodate requests for healthier options. For example, you can ask for steamed vegetables instead of french fries or request that your salad be made with a lighter dressing.

Consider sharing a dish: It can be tempting to order a large portion, but doing so can lead to overeating. Consider sharing a dish with a friend or family member or taking home leftovers for another meal.

By following these tips and being mindful of your choices, you can enjoy dining out while still maintaining a healthy diet. Remember, every little bit counts and every healthy choice you make is a step in the right direction.

Day 17: Managing Portion Sizes

Welcome to Day 17 of our healthy living journey! Today, we will be focusing on managing portion sizes.

Portion sizes are an important factor to consider when it comes to maintaining a healthy diet. Eating too much can lead to weight gain and other health issues, while eating too little can cause nutrient deficiencies. Finding the right balance is key.

Here are some tips to help you manage portion sizes:

Use smaller plates: Smaller plates can help you control your portion sizes and prevent overeating.

Measure your portions: Using measuring cups or a food scale can help you get a better sense of how much you are eating.

1. Practice mindful eating: Pay attention to your hunger and fullness levels and stop eating when you feel satisfied, rather than stuffed.
2. Read food labels: Look at serving sizes and pay attention to the number of servings in a package. This can help you better understand how much you are actually consuming.
3. Don't eat until you're stuffed: It takes time for your brain to register that you're full, so it's important to stop eating before you feel overly full.

By following these tips and being mindful of your portion sizes, you can make healthier choices and maintain a healthy weight. Remember, it's not about deprivation or restriction, but about finding a balance that works for you and your body.

Day 18: Ordering Special Requests and Modifications

Welcome to Day 18 of our customer service training series! Today, we will be discussing how to handle special requests and modifications from customers.

First, it's important to understand the difference between a special request and a modification. A special request is when a customer asks for something that is not normally offered or available. For example, a customer may request a vegetarian meal on a flight that only serves meat options. A modification, on the other hand, is when a customer wants to change something about their existing order. For example, a customer may want to change the size of their t-shirt or the color of their car.

Now that we have a clear understanding of the difference between special requests and modifications, let's go over how to handle them.

Listen carefully to the customer's request or modification: It's important to fully understand what the customer is asking for before trying to find a solution. Make sure to pay attention to their specific needs and preferences.

Determine if the request or modification is possible: Check to see if the request or modification is something that can be accommodated. If it is not possible, explain the situation to the customer and offer alternatives if possible.

1. Communicate any additional costs: If the request or modification will incur additional costs, make sure to clearly communicate this to the customer.
2. Confirm the request or modification: Once you have determined that the request or modification is possible and have communicated any additional costs, confirm the details with the customer to ensure that everyone is on the same page.
3. Follow up: Make sure to follow up with the customer to ensure that their request or modification was handled to their satisfaction.

Handling special requests and modifications can be challenging, but with clear communication and a customer-focused approach, you can provide excellent service to your customers.

Day 19: Dealing with Social Situations and Peer Pressure

Day 19: Dealing with Social Situations and Peer Pressure

Welcome to Day 19 of our customer service training series! Today, we will be discussing how to handle social situations and peer pressure when interacting with customers.

Social situations and peer pressure can be challenging to navigate, especially when you are in a customer-facing role. Here are some tips for handling these situations:

1. Remember your role: It's important to remember that as a customer service representative, your primary role is to provide excellent service to the customer. Don't be swayed by peer pressure or the desire to fit in with a group.

Stay professional: It's important to maintain a professional demeanor and not get caught up in any negative or inappropriate behavior.

2. Be empathetic: If a customer is upset or distressed, try to put yourself in their shoes and show empathy towards their situation.

3. Set boundaries: It's okay to set boundaries and say no if a customer is asking you to do something that goes against company policies or your own values.

4. Seek support: If you are feeling overwhelmed or uncomfortable in a social situation, it's okay to seek support from your manager or a colleague.

Dealing with social situations and peer pressure can be difficult, but by staying professional, being empathetic, setting boundaries, and seeking support when needed, you can handle these situations with grace and provide excellent customer service.

Day 20: Making Smart Choices at Fast Food Restaurants

Welcome to Day 20 of our customer service training series! Today, we will be discussing how to make smart choices when eating at fast food restaurants.

Eating at fast food restaurants can be convenient, but it's important to make healthy choices to maintain a balanced diet. Here are some tips for making smart choices at fast food restaurants:

Choose grilled or baked options instead of fried: Grilled or baked options are generally lower in fat and calories compared to fried options.

Look for options that are high in protein: Choose options that are high in protein, such as grilled chicken or a bean burrito, to keep you full and satisfied.

Choose water or low-fat milk instead of soda: Soda is high in sugar and calories, so opt for water or low-fat milk instead.

Opt for small sizes: Choose small sizes or "kids' meals" to help control portion sizes.

Avoid extra toppings: Extra toppings, such as cheese or sauces, can add extra calories and fat to your meal.

By following these tips, you can make healthier choices when eating at fast food restaurants. Remember, it's okay to treat yourself to fast food every once in a while, but it's important to maintain a balanced diet overall.

Day 21: Finding Healthy Options at Convenience Stores and Gas Stations

It can be challenging to find healthy options when you're on the go and only have access to convenience stores and gas stations. These places are often stocked with processed and sugary snacks, but there are still some choices you can make to stay on track with your health goals. Here are some tips for finding healthy options at convenience stores and gas stations:

Look for fresh fruits and vegetables: Many convenience stores and gas stations now offer a small selection of fresh produce, such as apples, bananas, and carrots. These can be a good source of fiber and nutrients, and can help to satisfy hunger without adding empty calories.

1. Choose whole grain options: Look for whole grain crackers, bread, and other grain-based snacks. These can be a good source of fiber and will help to keep you feeling full and satisfied.

2. Opt for protein-rich snacks: Hard-boiled eggs, nuts, and jerky can all be good options for satisfying protein. These snacks can help to keep you feeling full and satisfied between meals.

3. Avoid sugary drinks: Instead of soda or other sugary drinks, opt for water, unsweetened iced tea, or a low-sugar sports drink.
4. Look for healthy options in the cooler section: Many convenience stores and gas stations now offer healthy options such as Greek yogurt, hummus, and deli meats. These can be good choices for a quick, protein-rich snack.

Remember, it's okay to indulge in an occasional treat from a convenience store or gas station, but try to make healthy choices the majority of the time. With a little bit of planning and some smart choices, it's possible to maintain a healthy diet even when you're on the go.

Week 4: Staying on Track and Maintaining Progress

Week 4 of your journey is an important one, as it marks the midpoint of your program or goal. By now, you should have established some healthy habits and routines that are helping you stay on track and make progress toward your goal. However, it's important to keep in mind that progress doesn't always come in a straight line, and there may be setbacks or obstacles along the way. Here are some tips to help you stay on track and maintain your progress in week 4 and beyond:

Stay committed and consistent: Consistency is key when it comes to achieving any goal. Make sure you're sticking to your plan and following through on your commitments. Celebrate your progress: It's important to celebrate your successes and progress, no matter how small they may seem. This will help you stay motivated and keep pushing towards your goal.

1. Stay flexible: Don't be too rigid in your plan or approach. If something isn't working, be willing to adjust and adapt.
2. Seek support: Surround yourself with people who support your goals and can help you stay on track.

This could be friends, family, a coach, or a support group.

3. Stay motivated: Find ways to stay motivated and inspired, whether it's through reading success stories, listening to motivational podcasts, or setting small, achievable goals along the way.
4. Stay accountable: Consider finding an accountability partner or joining a group or program that helps keep you accountable to your goals.
5. Stay focused: It's easy to get sidetracked or distracted by other things. Make sure you're staying focused on your goal and not letting other things get in the way.

Remember, progress takes time and effort, and it's normal to have setbacks or challenges along the way. The key is to stay committed, consistent, and focused, and to keep pushing towards your goal.

Day 22: Meal Prep and Food Storage Techniques

Meal prep and food storage techniques can help you save time, and money, and eat healthier. Here are some tips for Day 22:

1. Plan your meals for the week: Decide what you want to eat for breakfast, lunch, dinner, and snacks for the next seven days. This will help you make a grocery list and avoid impulse buys.

2. Shop for ingredients: Make a list of the ingredients you need for your planned meals and stick to them when you go grocery shopping. If you want to save money and avoid packaging waste, think about buying in bulk.

3. Prep your ingredients: Wash and chop your fruits and vegetables as soon as you get home from the store. This will make it easier to grab and go when you're in a rush. You can also cook grains and proteins in advance, such as making a batch of quinoa or grilling chicken breasts.

4. Store food properly: Use airtight containers to store perishable items in the refrigerator. Consider using glass containers, which are more durable and better for the environment than plastic. You can also freeze pre-made meals or ingredients for future use.

5. Get creative with leftovers: Don't allow your leftovers to go to waste by being inventive with them. Get creative and repurpose them into new dishes. For example, you can turn leftover grilled chicken into a salad or use up extra vegetables in a stir-fry.

By following these meal prep and food storage techniques, you can save time, and money, and eat healthier throughout the week.

Day 23: Dealing with Cravings and Emotional Eating

Dealing with cravings and emotional eating can be a challenge, but there are strategies you can use to overcome them. Here are some tips for Day 23:

1. Identify the root cause of your cravings: Cravings can be triggered by physical hunger, boredom, stress, or emotional issues. Take a moment to reflect on what may be causing your cravings. Are you hungry, or are you seeking comfort or distraction?
2. Practice mindful eating: When you do have a craving, take a moment to pause and be present with your food. Engage your senses, savor the flavors and

textures, and pay attention to your body's hunger and fullness cues.

3. Find healthy ways to cope with emotions: Instead of turning to food to cope with negative emotions, try finding healthy ways to manage your feelings. This could include talking to a friend, going for a walk, or practicing relaxation techniques such as deep breathing or meditation.

4. Plan ahead: If you know you're prone to cravings at certain times of the day, have healthy snack options on hand. This can help you avoid reaching for unhealthy foods when you're feeling hungry or stressed.

5. Seek support: If you struggle with emotional eating or have a hard time managing your cravings, consider seeking support from a therapist or registered dietitian. They can help you identify the underlying causes of your cravings and develop healthy coping strategies.

By following these tips, you can learn to manage cravings and emotional eating healthily.

Day 24: Incorporating Mindfulness and Intuitive Eating

Incorporating mindfulness and intuitive eating into your daily routine can help you have a healthier relationship with food and your body. Here are some tips for Day 24:

1. Practice mindfulness: Mindfulness entails being conscious of the moment without passing judgment on it. When it comes to eating, this means being present with your food and paying attention to your body's hunger and fullness cues.
2. Eat without distractions: Turn off the TV, put away your phone, and focus on your meal. This will help you be more present and mindful while you eat.
3. Trust your body's hunger and fullness signals: Intuitive eating involves listening to your body's hunger and fullness cues and eating accordingly. This means eating when you're hungry and stopping when you're full, rather than following a strict diet or eating schedule.
4. Don't label foods as "good" or "bad": All foods can fit into a healthy diet, and labeling certain foods as "good" or "bad" can lead to an unhealthy relationship

with food. Instead, focus on nourishing your body with a variety of healthy, whole foods.

5. Let go of the diet mentality: Diets often focus on restrictions and rules, which can lead to a negative relationship with food. Instead of following a diet, try adopting a healthier, more sustainable way of eating that allows for flexibility and enjoyment.

By incorporating mindfulness and intuitive eating into your routine, you can develop a healthier relationship with food and your body.

Day 25: Finding Support and Encouragement

Finding support and encouragement can be an important part of making positive changes in your life, including improving your relationship with food and your body. Here are some tips for Day 25:

1. Reach out to friends and family: Having a supportive network of people can make a big difference when it comes to making changes in your life. Talk to your loved ones about your goals and ask for their support.

2. Join a support group: Consider joining a support group or online community of people who are

working towards similar goals. Sharing your experiences and receiving encouragement from others can be incredibly helpful.

3. Find a mentor or coach: If you're looking for more personalized support, consider finding a mentor or coach who can help you set and achieve your goals.

4. Practice self-compassion: Be kind to yourself and remember that it's okay to make mistakes. Instead of beating yourself up, try to be understanding and give yourself grace.

5. Celebrate your victories: Remember to celebrate your victories, no matter how small. This could be as simple as acknowledging that you made it through a tough day or as significant as reaching a major milestone.

By seeking out support and encouragement, you can increase your chances of success in making positive changes in your life.

Day 26: Making Lifestyle Changes for Long-Term Success

Making lifestyle changes can be a challenging but rewarding process. Here are some tips for Day 26 to help you achieve long-term success:

Start small: Rather than trying to make a lot of changes all at once, start with small, manageable steps. This will make the process more manageable and increase your chances of success.

Set specific, achievable goals: Rather than setting a vague goal like "lose weight," try setting specific, achievable goals like "exercise for 30 minutes three times a week" or "eat a serving of vegetables with every meal."

Make a plan: Once you've set your goals, make a plan for how you will achieve them. This could include scheduling workouts, meal planning, or finding accountability partners.

Be consistent: Consistency is key when it comes to making lifestyle changes. Try to make healthy habits a regular part of your routine rather than sporadic efforts.

Don't get discouraged: It's normal to have setbacks and challenges when making lifestyle changes. Don't get discouraged, and remember that progress is often made in small steps.

By starting small, setting specific goals, making a plan, and being consistent, you can increase your chances of long-term success in making positive lifestyle changes.

Day 27: Celebrating Progress and Setting New Goals

Today is a special day because it marks the end of my 27th day working towards my goals. It's a time to celebrate all of the progress I've made and to set new goals for the future.

To celebrate my progress, I'm going to take some time to reflect on all that I've accomplished over the past 27 days. This might include writing down a list of all of the tasks I've completed, reviewing any notes or journal entries I've made, and thinking about the challenges I've faced and how I've overcome them.

After taking some time to reflect on my progress, I'll set some new goals for the coming days and weeks. These goals might be related to my overall long-term goals, or they might be more specific and focused on specific tasks or areas of my life.

I'll make sure to be realistic and achievable with my new goals, but I'll also challenge myself to stretch and grow. Setting and working towards goals is an important way to stay motivated and focused, and it helps me to continue making progress in all areas of my life.

So today, I'll celebrate my progress and set new goals, knowing that each day is an opportunity to work towards becoming the best version of myself.

Day 28: Continuing the Journey Toward Better Health

Today is Day 28 of my journey toward better health, and I'm feeling motivated and determined to continue on this path.

Over the past 28 days, I've made several positive changes to my lifestyle and habits. I've been exercising regularly, eating a healthier diet, and making sure to get enough rest. These changes have already had a big impact on my overall well-being, and I'm feeling stronger and more energized as a result.

But I know that my journey towards better health is not over yet. There are still many challenges and obstacles ahead, and I need to stay focused and committed to my goals.

To help me stay on track, I'm going to continue to set small, achievable goals for myself. I'll track my progress and celebrate my successes along the way. And I'll remind myself that every day is a new opportunity to make healthy choices and work towards my goals.

I'm excited to see what the next 28 days (and beyond) bring as I continue on this journey toward better health.

Conclusion

The Benefits of a Diabetes Diet Plan for Weight Loss

A diabetes diet plan can be a helpful tool for anyone looking to lose weight, particularly those with type 2 diabetes. There are several benefits to following a diabetes diet plan for weight loss, including:

Improved blood sugar control: A diabetes diet plan focuses on foods that can help stabilize blood sugar levels and reduce the risk of high and low blood sugar spikes. This can be especially beneficial for those with type 2 diabetes, as maintaining stable blood sugar levels can help prevent long-term complications such as nerve damage and kidney disease.

Weight loss: By following a diabetes diet plan, you may be able to lose weight and improve your overall health. Losing weight can help reduce the risk of developing type 2 diabetes or help manage the condition if you already have it.

Increased energy levels: A healthy diabetes diet plan can help improve your energy levels by providing your body with the nutrients it needs to function properly. This can help you feel more energized and motivated to be active and pursue your weight loss goals.

Improved mood: Eating a healthy, balanced diet can also help improve your mood and reduce the risk of developing mental health conditions such as depression and anxiety.

Overall, following a diabetes diet plan can be an effective way to lose weight and improve your overall health. It's important to work with a healthcare provider or registered dietitian to create a plan that meets your individual needs and goals.

Tips for Sustaining Progress and Maintaining a Healthy Lifestyle

Tips for Sustaining Progress and Maintaining a Healthy Lifestyle

Sustaining progress and maintaining a healthy lifestyle can be challenging, but several tips can help you stay on track:

Set achievable goals: It's important to set realistic, achievable goals for yourself. This will help you stay motivated and focused on the progress you're making.

Track your progress: Keep track of your progress, whether it's through a journal, a fitness tracker, or simply by checking in with yourself regularly. Seeing the progress you've made can be a powerful motivator.

Find a support system: Surround yourself with people who support and encourage your healthy lifestyle. These might be close friends, relatives, or a support network. Having a strong support system can help you stay motivated and accountable.

Incorporate physical activity into your routine: Regular physical activity is an important part of maintaining a healthy lifestyle. Try to find activities that you enjoy and that fit into your schedule.

Eat a balanced diet: Focus on eating a variety of nutrient-dense foods, including fruits, vegetables, whole grains, lean proteins, and healthy fats. As much as you can, stay away from processed, sugary, and high-fat foods.

Maintain your hydration: Water consumption is crucial for a healthy body. Sleep for 7-9 hours per night, per day.

Get enough sleep: Getting enough sleep is crucial for maintaining good physical and mental health. Per day, aim for at least 8 to 8 ounces of water.

By following these tips, you can help sustain your progress and maintain a healthy lifestyle over the long term.